Mediterranean Diet

Mediterranean Diet: The Ultimate Beginner's Guide & Cookbook To Mediterranean Diet - Meal Plan Recipes To Lose Weight & Lower Risk of Heart Disease +14 Day Meal Plan, 40+ Easy & Proven Heart Healthy Recipes

By *Simone Jacobs*

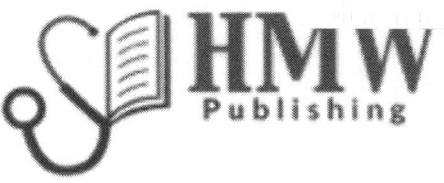

For more great books visit:

HMWPublishing.com

Get another book for Free

I want to thank you for purchasing this book and offer you another book (just as long and valuable as this book), "Health & Fitness Mistakes You Don't Know You're Making", completely free.

Visit the link below to signup and receive it:

www.hmwpublishing.com/gift

In this book, I will break down the most common health & fitness mistakes, you are probably committing right now, and I will reveal how you can easily get in the best shape of your life!

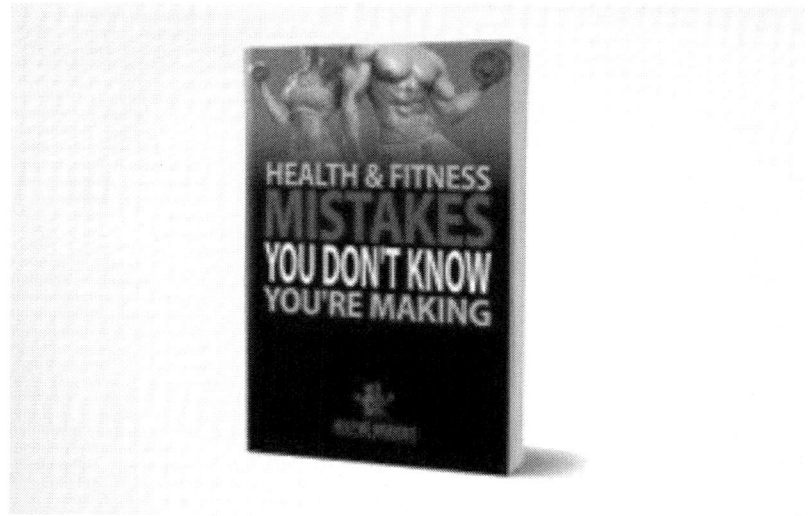

In addition to this valuable gift, you will also have an opportunity to get our new books for free, enter giveaways, and receive other valuable emails from me. Again, visit the link to sign up:

www.hmwpublishing.com/gift

Table of Contents

INTRODUCTION

I want to thank you and congratulate you for purchasing the *"The Ultimate Beginner's Guide To Mediterranean Diet And Meal Plan PLUS Recipes"* book.

This book contains proven steps and strategies on how you can lose weight and become more healthy without having to go on a real diet. You'll also discover how you can eat the filling and delicious meals. Moreover, you'll learn the advantages of packing your meals with veggies, fruits, nuts, legumes, and more. Likewise, you will also learn some helpful tips on how you can succeed in adopting the Mediterranean diet. Lastly, we even provide you with a sample meal plan and Mediterranean-friendly recipes, which you can get started right away! Thanks again for purchasing this book, I hope you enjoy it !

Also, before you get started, I recommend you **joining our email newsletter** to receive updates on any upcoming new book releases or promotions. You can sign-up for free, and as a bonus, you will receive a free gift. Our *"Health & Fitness Mistakes You Don't Know You're Making"* book! This book has been written to demystify, expose the top do's and don'ts and to finally equip you with the information you need to get in the best shape of your life. Due to the overwhelming amount of mis-information and lies told by magazines and self-proclaimed "gurus", it's becoming harder and harder to get reliable information to get in shape. As opposed to having to go through dozens of biased, unreliable and un-trustworthy sources to get your health & fitness information. Everything you need to help you has been broken down in this book for you to easily follow and to immediately get results to achieve your desired fitness goals in the shortest amount of time.

Once again, to join our free email newsletter and to receive a free copy of this valuable book, please visit the link and signup now: **www.hmwpublishing.com/gift**

CHAPTER 1: WHAT IS THE MEDITERRANEAN DIET?

The Mediterranean is not a real diet or similar to the many diets that involves eliminating carbs, eating a specific ratio of macronutrients, reducing the amount of a certain food in your meals, or eliminating a certain food.

Rather, this diet is a lifestyle that involves eating food based on the traditional recipes, beverages, and dishes of the countries surrounding the Mediterranean Sea, along with physical activities, meals with family and friends, and drinking wine in moderation with the meals. To put it simply, the Mediterranean diet is adopting the cooking style, cuisine, and eating habits of people from the Mediterranean.

The main objective of this diet is to "eat like a Greek", which has been noted as one of the healthiest eating habits in the world. It generally involves:

- Planning your meals to consist mainly of legumes, nuts, whole grains, fruits, vegetables, and other foods that are plant-based;

- Using canola, olive oil, and other healthy oils and fats instead of using butter;

- Using spices and herbs to add flavor to foods instead of using salt;

- Consuming red meat not more than 1 to 2 times monthly;

- Consuming poultry and fish at least twice a week

- Drinking wine moderately

- Getting plenty of exercise and other physical activities

Together with eating healthy, the Mediterranean diet also gives importance on making delicious and flavorful dishes and meals. If you are new to this diet, you might think that eating like a Greek and the Mediterranean cooking-style is a complex. Well, nothing is easy when you are just starting to learn how to do it, no matter what kind of diet you choose to do.

The fabulous thing about this diet, once you decided to adopt it and make the changes, it's quite simple, as well as fun. You will find that there are thousands of natural, healthy, and scrumptious dishes. It's a great way to improve your health and lose weight, without having to sacrifice the taste of your food.

A Little Bit of History about the Mediterranean Diet

The roots and the origin of this diet is in the Mediterranean basin, a place that is also referred to by the historians as "the cradle of history." It is where the whole history of the ancient world happened within its geographical borders. To be more specific, the Mediterranean diet was based on the traditional foods that the people of countries like Greece and Italy used to eat back in the 1960s.

Although the Mediterranean diet is a modern and just a recently promoted nutritional recommendation, this healthy lifestyle is as old as the civilizations that lived in the Nile River, a region where ancient, yet advanced civilization arose. Along with the progress of the cultures, customs, languages, religions, thinking, history and lifestyle that flourished in the region, the eating habit of the people there became and the melting pot of various cuisines.

The actual story of the Mediterranean diet is lost in time. The passing of time has changed the diet in various and many ways possible. However, the traditional foods remained, and vegetables remained its main ingredient.

The Mediterranean diet that we know today is the result of a long history, various traditions intertwining with one another, the combination of multiple rich cuisines of the countries in the Mediterranean region, and the addition of modern food. Although the original diet has changed over the course of history, the present Mediterranean diet closely resembles the original diet.

Currently, the Mediterranean diet has been discovered as an eating habit that's effective in helping people improve their health and excess lose weight, at the same time eating flavorful, rich, pure dishes –an eating lifestyle has preserved the traditions and customs of the Mediterranean region.

How Does the Mediterranean Diet Work?

We are what we eat. What we eat dictates how healthy and how long our bodies will live. The foods we eat have direct and profound effects on our health. Why is it important to eat healthily? Consuming foods that are rich in vitamins and minerals help prevent various diseases, such as hypertension, obesity, diabetes, and helps keep the cells and your body in top shape.

The Mediterranean was initially been discovered and recognized as a healthy eating habit as early as the 1950s by Dr. Ancel Benjamin Keys from the University of Minnesota School of Power. Keys laid the foundations of the Mediterranean diet that we know now. He also hypothesized that various eating habits have different effects on health. The discovery of the numerous health benefits of the diet is also thanks to him. He was the first person to point out that the Mediterranean diet helps decrease cardiovascular disease.

Keys led the famous "Seven Countries Study" that

documented the relationship between lifestyle nutrition and cardiovascular disease. It proved that the many health benefits a person could reap with the Mediterranean diet. Furthermore, the study revealed that people on the Mediterranean diet had very low cholesterol, which means a lower risk of developing coronary heart disease. The findings of the showed that this health benefit is due to a diet that is primarily composed of bread, pasta, spices and herbs, vegetables, fruits, olive oil, and other plant-based food.

From Dr. Keys' pioneering study, numerous studies and researchers have followed to determine the relationship between dietary habits and chronic diseases. These studies have corroborated the health benefits of the Mediterranean diet. Many of the clinical studies and trials have shown the following health benefits of eating like a Greek.

- Reduce the risk of cardiovascular disease and metabolic syndrome

- Decrease belly or abdominal fat

- Increase the levels of high-density lipoprotein (HDL)

or healthy fat

- Decrease the levels of triglycerides

- Lower blood pressure, and

- Decrease the levels of glucose in the blood

However, the various studies emphasize that eating like a Greek by itself will not produce the health benefits mentioned above. The total calories consumed and the amount of exercise done by a person affects the individual's health as well. They advise that along with a healthy eating habit; one must also exercise or engage in physical activities. Dr. Keys stressed that the Mediterranean diet is not just a diet - it is a healthy lifestyle.

By 1993, the European Office of the World Health Organization, the Harvard School of Public Health, and Oldways officially introduced the classic Mediterranean in, in Cambridge Massachusetts. Their presentation included the Mediterranean Diet Pyramid visual representation. It explained the most up-to-date nutrition study that characterizes the healthy, traditional Mediterranean diet. It also described the original Mediterranean Diet pyramid that was made based on the dietary habits of countries like Greece and Italy in the 1960s, a time when, even though the medical services were limited, the adult chronic diseases to be the lowest and the life expectancy was the highest.

From that basic pyramid model, it was updated to include the other vital elements, which consists of the following components:

- Daily exercise

- Sharing meals with friends and family, and

- Nurturing a sincere appreciation for eating healthy and delicious food

On November 2008, the Mediterranean diet pyramid was updated again to include the latest research findings. The herbs and spices used in various Mediterranean cuisines were added. The placement of the fish and shellfish was changed to recognize the benefits of consuming them at least twice per week. Finally, a consensus from Scientific Advisory Board updated the Mediterranean diet to focus on more plant-based foods in healthy eating - this is the Mediterranean diet that many people now enjoy.

CHAPTER 2: HOW TO LIVE LONGER

As shown by the findings of the "Seven Countries Study" lead by Dr. Ancel Keys, people who ate a diet the comprised mostly of fish, beans, grains, fruit, and vegetables were among the healthiest.

An Incredibly Delicious Way to Lose Weight and Be Healthy

The Mediterranean diet is among the world's oldest diet. It is also among the world's most effective weight loss diet and the healthiest. But how does the food we eat affect our health, for better or for worse? Let's take a look, shall we?

Seeds and Nuts

They are high in micronutrients, which are vital for the proper functioning of the body. They are mostly made up of monounsaturated fat or MUFA. Research has shown that MUFA helps burn fat in the body, even when a person is not doing anything. Seeds and nuts are also packed with omega-e fatty acids, which the body cannot make on their own.

Hence, you need to get them through the food you eat. They are also a good source of magnesium, protein, and vitamin E.

Fruit

Don't grab foods that are packed with unhealthy artificial sweeteners. If you are hungry between meals, grab a fruit instead. Fruits contain fructose, a natural sugar that is also found in veggies and root crops, which is a good source of energy and satisfy your cravings for sweet. Unlike artificial sweeteners, fructose does not increase calorie intake, store excess calories into fat, or increase levels of insulin.

Spices and Herbs

They add aroma and flavor to food. They also contain natural chemicals that help remove toxins that store fat from the body, decrease body inflammation that causes weight gain, break down fat cells, lower blood sugar levels, decrease cravings for sugary and fatty foods, and increase metabolism.

As they add natural aroma, color, and flavor to dishes, spices and herbs reduce and eliminates adding unhealthy fat sugar, and salt in recipes.

Wine

Wine contains Resveratrol, antioxidants that help increase metabolism for one and a half hours after enjoying a glass, which aids in weight loss. Studies found out that Resveratrol reduces fat in the liver, decrease body inflammation, improve cell function, lower blood sugar and insulin levels.

Whole Grains

Complex carbohydrates are needed for the proper functioning of the body, as well as help it lose weight, so don't believe the hype – reducing your carbohydrate intake won't give your body any benefits. A diet low in carbohydrates depletes your body with its much-needed carbs, notably its purer form – glucose, the body's primary source of energy. Glucose fuels the immune system, muscles, heart, brain, and other fundamental bodily function.

If you have tried lowering your carb intake and then you know that it comes with feeling miserable and irritable. It's your body telling you that you are not getting enough glucose or energy. Even if you are trying to lose excess weight, the body needs about 45 to 65 percent of complex carbohydrates. Studies show that people who get 64 percent of their daily calorie need form complex carbohydrates are fitter, compared to those who ate less.

Seafood

They are high in omega-3 fatty acids that help increase the body's sensitivity to blood sugar. Consuming shellfish and fish at least twice a week increases as well as increase metabolism by up to 400 calories and the body's fat-burning ability.

Beans

These are packed with both soluble and insoluble fiber. Similar to vegetables, soluble fibers dissolve with the liquids in the stomach to form a gel. This gell formation helps aids you in feeling fuller longer. Insoluble fiber, on the other hand, absorbs water, adding more bulk to your digestive system.

Vegetables

Almost every person eats the same kinds of food every day. The key to a healthier body and weight loss is to consume more vegetables. Veggies are bulky with fewer calories. They are packed with micronutrients – antioxidants, phytochemicals, vitamins, and minerals that the body needs. Studies show that if a person's body is low in micronutrients, even just moderately little, the body's metabolism will slow down because it is not getting enough B vitamins, magnesium, and other nutrients. When the metabolism slows down, the body is not burning fat.

As you know, the human body is made up of around 60 to 70 percent water. When you are dehydrated, even just mildly dehydrated, the body will stop functioning correctly, which includes slowing down of metabolism, digestion, and fat burning.

Eating veggies ensure you get the right amount of water because they are made up of 90 percent water. Furthermore, these green leafy vegetables are packed with fiber that fights off craving and hunger which aids you to feel fuller longer.

Greek Yogurt

These ready to eat food are packed with more protein an ounce than any other ready to eat food. Consuming Greek yogurt reduces cravings, prevent overeating, and stabilize blood sugar level, curb hunger, and increase feelings of fullness.

Researchers have shown that eating Greek yogurt ensures that the body gets the right amount of good bacteria. When the body has a healthy balance of good bacteria, it enhances the metabolism of the body and burns fat faster.

Moreover, they are rich in calcium, minerals that are good for the bones. Calcium also helps hasten fat burning. However, researchers about this stress that it is not as simple as taking a calcium supplement. They added that along with calcium, a person must consume enough protein at the same time to reap its weight loss benefits successfully. Protein without calcium will also not do the trick.

Olive Oil

This oil is a powerful and effective stimulant for weight loss. Its scent alone will help you feel fuller, making you eat less, and fewer calories. Olive oil is 75 percent monounsaturated fat or MUFA, the highest amount of any oil or food. Studies show that MUFA burns fat even if the person is not doing anything at all. Furthermore, studies show that consuming 1 spoonful of olive oil during breakfast increases fat oxidation and increases the body's ability to use fat as fuel or energy.

Furthermore, olive oil is condensed with oleic acid. This oil is a compound that helps halt the feeling of hunger; which also makes you feel fuller for a longer time. Additionally, the oleic acid helps lower blood sugar level and control insulin.

The Health Benefits of the Mediterranean Diet

So what do you get when you combine all the health benefits of the food mentioned above? You will the numerous health benefits below.

Improves fertility

If you are trying to conceive, then a Mediterranean diet will increase your chances of having a baby. According to a study published in the Journal of Fertility and Sterility, people on the Mediterranean diet had more chances of getting pregnant via intra-cytoplasmic sperm injection (ICSI) or in vitro fertilization (IVF).

Maintains healthy dentures

According to the findings published in the Molecular Oral Microbiology, marine and plant omega -3 fatty acids have strong anti-bacterial properties against numerous oral pathogens, keeping the teeth healthy.

Keeps the eyes healthy

People on the Mediterranean diet have a lesser risk of developing macular degeneration, particularly in older people. A study by the Centre for Eye Research Australia (CERA) revealed that consuming at least 100 ml of olive oil weekly reduces the risk of developing poor eyesight.

Healthier babies

It's vital that a mom-to-be consumes fish and seafood during the third trimester of her pregnancy. Studies show that a Mediterranean diet reduces the risk of spina bifida in babies, a congenital disability characterized by spinal cord deformity. This healthy diet also reduces low birth weight in infants. Moreover, children whose mothers who ate at least 2 servings of fish weekly have higher intelligence.

Healthier Lungs

The Mediterranean diet helps prevent, and also protect, children from childhood asthma, wheezing, allergic rhinitis, and asthma-like symptoms. Adults who have been consuming this healthy diet for a long time have less incidence of asthma. Moreover, long-term consumption of Mediterranean diet reduces the risk of chronic obstructive pulmonary disease, chronic bronchitis, or emphysema.

Alleviates rheumatoid arthritis

People with rheumatoid arthritis who adopted the Mediterranean diet experienced reduced inflammation, improved vitality, and increased physical function.

Prevents Parkinson's disease

Because the Mediterranean diet is packed with healthy fats, low in saturated fat, and moderate in alcohol consumption, it stops and protects the brain against Parkinson's disease.

Prevents Alzheimer's disease

Studies show that together with regular exercise or being active, the Mediterranean will help decrease the risk of Alzheimer's disease by 48 percent. The main component of the diet – using non-animal fat, complex carbohydrates, and fiber – protects against cognitive decline linked to age, as well as vascular and degenerative cognitive problems.

Keeps the blues away

Legumes, fish, nuts, vegetables, fruits, and other vital nutrients are linked to a better mindset ad happier mood, thus preventing depression.

Aids weight loss management efforts

The Mediterranean diet stresses on consuming monounsaturated fats or MUFA-rich instead of saturated fat. MUFA helps burn fat even when a person is not doing anything, which helps the body lose excessive weight gain and improves glycemic control. Moreover, various studies reveal that the Mediterranean diet helps lower the occurrence of obesity in both women and men, which prevents weight gain and promotes weight loss.

Protects from diabetes

A study shows rich in omega-3 essential fatty acid prevents insulin resistance, which decreases the risk of diabetes.

Lowers cholesterol, blood pressure levels, and risk of heart disease

The Mediterranean diet, a diet high in nuts, monounsaturated fatty acids, and vegetables, is rich in omega-3 fatty acids, folate, and vitamin C and E, which is shown to reduce blood coagulation and inflammation of the heat, hypertension, insulin resistance, blood pressure levels, and heart disease.

Fights certain cancers

Studies on the benefits of the Mediterranean diet show that the Mediterranean diet reduces the risk of stomach cancer or gastric adenocarcinoma. Moreover, it also showed that consuming as little as 10 teaspoons of olive oil prevents the development of breast cancer in women. Additionally, olive oil has been shown to inhibit and fight cancer tumors. Other studies show that a diet high in fruits, vegetables, whole grains, and fish decrease the risk of skin cancer or carcinoma.

Fights certain chronic diseases

Because the Mediterranean diet is high in plant-based foods, has a healthy unsaturated and saturated fat ratio, it helps lower the risk of chronic diseases, including obesity, hypercholesterolemia or high cholesterol levels in the blood, diabetes, and hypertension.

Together with exercise or regular physical activity and not smoking, research suggests that the Mediterranean diet helps lower diabetes by up to 90 percent, coronary heart disease by up to80 percent, and stroke by up to 70 percent.

Improves cognitive function

The diet is packed with whole grains, fish, fruits, and olive oil, foods that protect the brain from cognitive problems and damage.

Lengthens life

Overall, the Mediterranean diet combines the all of the health benefits of delicious and healthy foods in one. By increasing the amount of the good stuff and reducing the amount of the food that are less healthy, it will significantly improve your health. At the same time, it reduces the risk of Parkinson's disease, Alzheimer's disease, cancer, cardiovascular disease, and other major chronic diseases.

Over the centuries, since the discovery of the possible health benefits of the Mediterranean diet by Dr. Keys, numerous studies and researchers have then and again provided evidence to back them up. So if you are ready to start the journey to a healthier you, then read on.

Chapter 3: The Start of a Journey to Health

Although the Mediterranean diet is not a real diet, it has 9 protocols or basic rules according to the 2,000 calorie daily needs for men and 1,500 calories per day for women.

Alcohol

If you are not a drinker, then there is no need to start drinking alcoholic drinks. Interestingly, however, men who drink a healthy 1 to 2 glasses a day lowers the risk of heart attack.

How Much Can I consume on the Mediterranean diet?

 If you drink, then keep it to 2 drinks a day if you are a man and to 1 glasses 1 day if you are a woman.

Note that 1 drink is equal to 1 ounce of hard liquor, such as vodka, whiskey, gin, etc., or 4 to 5 ounces of wine. Moreover, do not save up all the alcohol to drink it all at once.

Remember that the limit is 1-2 glasses daily.

Meats

The Mediterranean diet involves eating less meat, both red and white. A typical diet suggests that a person should consume 4 ounces of meat a day and eat red meat only once a week.

How Much Can I consume on the Mediterranean diet?

A man should eat less than 3.9 ounces and a woman 3.25 ounces. However, if you are following the strict Mediterranean diet, then follow the pyramid guidelines below.

Dairy

Dairy, as well as dairy products, is not an essential food of the Mediterranean diet. Usually, when milk is part of a recipe, it is generally in the form of yogurt or cheese.

How much is in the Mediterranean diet?

Men should consume less than 7.2 ounces and women less than 6.9 ounces.

Fats and Oils

Mentioned a couple of times earlier, the Mediterranean diet stresses on consuming more monounsaturated fats, which you should consume primarily from olive oil. However, you can also use other oils that are high in monounsaturated fats, such as canola oil. On this matter, many claims that grapeseed oil is better than canola oil or olive oil.

However, the key is to decrease or to eliminate the use of highly saturated oils or fat, such as lard, coconut oil, shortening, palm kernel oil, butter, or any hydrogenated oil.

How Much Can I consume on the Mediterranean diet?

Instead of calculating your daily consumption of fats, both women and men should consume 60 percent of unsaturated fat than saturated fat.

Fish

On the Mediterranean diet, you will eat more fish and less meat.

What to Do If You Don't Like Fish

Start with the kind that you like or familiar with, then slowly try the kind that you want less and less familiar with.

Fish are a better source of protein than meat. They also have lower fat content and seafood contains good fats, including omega-3 fatty acids, which are famous for their ability to reduce heart disease and stroke. Moreover, several studies indicate that consuming food rich in omega-3 fatty acids prevent certain types of cancer, as well as help alleviate problems with heart rhythm.

How Much Can I consume on the Mediterranean diet?

Men should eat at least 1 ounce and women should eat at least 0.75 ounces daily. Please note, there have been concerns about mercury contamination lately. However, this does not mean that you can't consume seafood. You just need to be careful. The advantages of eating fish greatly outweigh the risk of contaminants. The Centers for Disease Control and Prevention recommends avoiding fish with more than 1.0 ppm (parts per billion) of mercury. Check the list of fish that you need to avoid. I have included a file on the subsequent pages of this book. It gives you.

Cereals and Grains

On the Mediterranean diet, whole grains are high. However, if you are used to eating "white" starches, such as pasta, white rice, and white bread, then slowly shift to whole grains. You can begin with eating "light" whole-wheat bread, then slowly move to whole grain bread. If eating white rice, substitute any recipe that calls for it with brown rice. Replacing white rice with brown rice instantly increases your fiber consumption. You can also replace real potatoes with sweet potatoes and yams. Always choose whole-grain cereals.

How Much Can I consume on the Mediterranean diet?

Men should at least 10.4 ounces and women at least 8.9 ounces of cereals and grains daily.

Nuts and Fruits

Nuts are perfect as snacks. They contain plenty of calories, but these calories come mainly from monounsaturated fat or MUFA, which are suitable fats that help the body lose weight. In fact, studies show that if you eat 2 ounces of nuts instead of cookies, you will not gain any weight even though the nuts contain more calories than the cookies.

Fruits are the perfect sweet snacks. They satisfy your sweet tooth cravings without adding artificial sweeteners and additives into your diet. Pack your pantry and refrigerator with pears, apples, oranges, and more. Enjoying your fruits are juice is acceptable on the Mediterranean diet, but it's better to eat them since it will preserve their fiber content.

How Much Can I consume on the Mediterranean diet?

Men should eat about 8.9 ounces daily while women should consume approximately 7.7 ounces a day.

Legumes

There are different kinds of vegetables that you can choose from to include in your diet. They are an excellent source of fiber and an excellent source of alternative protein. Legumes are also versatile. You can add them as an ingredient in your salads, soups, or main course recipes, or serve them as a side dish.

How Much Can I consume on the Mediterranean diet?

Men should consume about 2.1 ounces, and women should eat approximately 1.75 ounces daily.

Vegetables

Veggies are the most important and the major component of the Mediterranean diet. There is no way you can eat too many vegetables. You can eat a lot and still be within your recommended daily calorie intake. They help you feel full faster and longer.

One great way to increase your consumption of vegetables is to include them in your lunch and snack. Pile your favorite sandwich with onion, peppers, tomatoes, cucumbers, lettuce, and virtually anything you desire.

What to Do If you do not Like Veggies

Similar to fish, you can begin with the ones that you like. Think of all the veggies that you have already eaten and kept them on hand. Then slowly explore and add the ones that are less familiar to you.

How Much Can I consume on the Mediterranean diet?

Men should eat at least 10.8 ounces and women at least 8.9 ounces a day.

The Mediterranean Diet Pyramid

The Mediterranean diet follows a food pyramid. Use the guide below to plan your dishes according to what you can eat daily or weekly.

Daily Menu

Non-starchy vegetables (4-8 servings)

A serving size is:

- 1 cup raw vegetables

- One-half cup cooked vegetables

Non-starchy vegetables include all plants, except winter squash, peas, corn, and potatoes.

Healthy fats (4-6 servings)

A serving size is:

- 1 teaspoon olive or canola oil

- 2 teaspoons light margarine

- 1 tablespoon regular salad dressing

- 2 tablespoons light salad dressing (made with 1

teaspoon regular mayonnaise, 5 olives, and 1/8 avocado)

Whole grains and starchy vegetables (4-6 servings)

A serving size is:

- 1 slice bread, whole-wheat

- One-half cup corn, peas, potatoes, or winter squash

- 1/2 of a large-sized whole-grain bun

- 1 small-sized whole-grain roll

- 6 inches whole-wheat pita

- 6 whole-grain crackers

- One-half cup cooked whole-grain cereal

- One-half cup cooked barley, whole-wheat pasta, or brown rice

Fruits (2-4 servings)

A serving size is:

- One-half cup juice

- 1 small-sized fresh fruit

- One-fourth cup dried fruit

Always choose whole fruits, because they contain fiber and other nutrients. If you are using canned fruits, want the variety with no sugar or low sugar added. Consume no more than 8 ounces a day of fruit juices since even the unsweetened types are high in sugar.

Legumes and nuts (1-3 servings)

Aim for a 1-2 serving of nuts daily and 1-2 serving of vegetables daily.

A serving size is:

- 2 tablespoons sesame or sunflower seeds

- 1 tablespoon peanut butter

- 7 to 8 walnuts

- 20 peanuts

- 12 to 15 almonds

- One-fourth cup baked or refried beans, fat-free

- One-half cup kidney, lentils, navy beans, split peas, pinto, soy, black, or garbanzo beans

Weekly Menu

Fish (2-3 servings)

A serving is 3 ounces or about the size of a deck of cards.

Dairy (1-3 servings)

A serving is:

- 1 cup of light yogurt, non-fat yogurt, or skim milk

- 10 ounces low-fat cheese

You can use soy cheese, soy milk, or soy yogurt instead.

Poultry (1-3 servings)

A serving is 3 ounces or about the size of a deck of cards. This is optional; you can opt not to add any poultry to your Mediterranean diet.

Monthly Menu

Eggs

You can eat as much as 4 egg yolks weekly. On the other

hand, you can eat as much egg whites as you want.

Sweets

You can eat once a week or 3 to 4 times monthly.

Red meats (veal, lamb, and beef)

You can eat once a week or 3 to 4 times monthly.

Substitutions

If you want to replace a recipe ingredient with an ingredient that you like, then be sure to use an amount with the same or similar calorie count as the original. For example, you want to replace chicken with a salmon. A 2.6 ounces chicken has 176 calories, so you must replace it with 3 ounces of salmon, which contains 177 calories.

If you would like to substitute green beans with tomatoes, then replace 3/4 cup of green beans containing 26 calories with 1 cup cherry tomatoes containing 26 calories.

If you prefer strawberries instead of peaches, 2/3 cup peaches contain 44 calories, which you can replace with 1 cup strawberries containing 47 calories.

Important Reminders

The Mediterranean pyramid is a reliable guide for most adults. However, children, pregnant women, and people with special dietary needs may need nutritional supplements on a diet. In most circumstances, these special dietary needs can be accommodated on the Mediterranean diet.

CHAPTER 4: THE MEDITERRANEAN DIET FOOD LIST

Are you ready to fill your pantry and fridge? Here is the list of the standard ingredients of the Mediterranean diet. Use this guide to plan your dishes and meals.

Vegetables

Zucchini Squash	Yellow Squash	Tomatoes	Squash
Spinach	Shallots	Peppers	Peas
Peas	Onions	Lettuce	Leeks
Green Onions	Green Beans	Eggplant	Eggplant
Cucumbers	Collard Greens	Celery	Cabbage
Button Mushrooms	Brussels Sprouts	Beets	Bean sprouts
Asparagus	Acorn Squash		

Legumes

White Kidney Bean (Fazolia Bean, Cannellini Bean)	Sugar Snap Peas (Snap Peas)
Soy Bean (Soya Bean, Edamame)	Snow Peas (Chinese Pea)
Runner Bean (Italian Flat Bean)	Red Kidney Beans (Red Beans, Mexican Beans)
Pinto Beans	Okra
Navy Beans (Yankee Bean, Boston Bean, Boston Navy Bean)	Lima Beans
Lentils	Green Beans (String Bean, Haricot Verts)
Great Northern Bean	Garbanzo Beans (Chick Peas)
Fava Bean (Windsor Bean, Broad Bean, English Bean, Butter Bean)	English Peas

Black Beans (Spanish Black Beans, Turtle Beans, Mexican Black Beans)	

Nuts and Fruits

Walnuts	Sunflower Seeds	Raspberries	Pumpkin Seeds
Pistachios	Pine Nuts	Pecans	Pears
Peanuts	Peaches	Oranges	Nectarines
Macadamia Nuts	Hazelnuts	Grapes	Cranberries
Cereals and Grains	Cashews	Blueberries	Blackberries
Bananas	Apples	Almonds	

Substitutions

Instead of...	Choose...
White Rice	Brown Rice or Wild Rice
White Bread	Whole Wheat Bread
Special K	Cheerios
Rice Krispies	Kashi GoLean Crunch
Regular Pasta	Whole Wheat Pasta or Quinoa Pasta
Pizza Dough	Whole Wheat Pizza Dough
Grits	Oatmeal
Fruit Loops	Life Cereal
English Muffin	Whole Wheat English Muffin
Corn Flakes	Bran Flakes
Corn	Beans or Lentils
Bagel	Whole Wheat Bagel
Apple Jacks	Kashi Cinnamon Harvest

Fish

Fish	Omega-3 fats per 4 ounces serving	Mercury parts per billion (ppm)
Anchovy	2,055 mg	<0.05
Wild Salmon	1,043 mg	<0.05
Trout	935 mg	0.07
Shrimp	315 mg	<0.05
Scallops	365 mg	<0.05
Sardines	982 mg	<0.05
Oysters	688 mg	<0.05
Mussels	782 mg	<0.15
Light Tuna	270 mg	0.12
Farmed Salmon	2,648 mg	<0.05
Farmed Catfish	177 mg	<0.05
Crab	351 mg	0.09
Clams	284 mg	<0.05
Atlantic Mackerel	1,203 mg	0.05

Atlantic Herring	2,014 mg	<0.05
Atlantic Cod	158 mg	0.1

Fats and Oils

Good choices	Use carefully	Avoid
Tahini (sesame seed butter)		
Sesame oil	Spreads like Smart Balance Light and	Vegetable shortening
Safflower oil	Promise Light	Stick margarine
Peanut butter	Mayonnaise	Lard
Olive Oil	Coconut milk	Foods containing palm kernel oil
Grapeseed oil	Butter	Foods containing hydrogenated oils
Canola Oil	Avocados	Coconut oil

Dairy

Yogurt Cheese	Yogurt	Ricotta Cheese
Reduced-fat White Cheddar	Reduced-fat Cheeses	Pecorino
Parmigiano	Mozzarella	Monterey Jack Cheese
Milk	Low-fat White Cheddar	Evaporated Milk
Cream Cheese - Fat-Free	Cream Cheese	Buttermilk
Butter	Blue Cheese	

The Mediterranean Diet Shopping Guide

Oils

Olive Oil	Extra-virgin olive oil

Vinegar

Balsamic	Red wine	White wine

Spices and dried herbs

Rosemary	Red and white wine	Parsley	Oregano	Ginger
Garlic	Fennel seed	Dill	Cumin	Coriander
Cloves	Cinnamon	Cayenne pepper	Basil	

Seafood and Meat

Clams	Cod	Crab meat
Halibut	Mussels	Salmon
Scallops	Shrimp	Tilapia
Tuna	Chicken breast (1-2 times weekly)	Chicken thighs (1-2 times weekly)
Lean red meat (1-2 times monthly)		

Packaged and Canned

Olives	Canned Tomatoes	Canned tuna

Canned and Dried Beans

Navy beans	Lentils	Kidney beans
Chickpeas	Cannellini beans	Black beans

Whole Grains

Whole-wheat couscous	Whole-wheat bread or pita	Whole-grain pasta
Whole-grain crackers	Quinoa	Polenta
Oats	Faro	Bulgur
Brown rice	Barley	

Seeds and Nuts

Walnuts	Sunflower seeds	Sesame seeds
Pine nuts	Hazelnuts	Cashews
Almonds		

Refrigerated

Plain or Greek yogurt	Low-fat milk	Eggs

Cheese

Ricotta	Parmesan	Mozzarella	Goat cheese
Feta	Cream cheese		

Produce

Zucchini	Tomatoes	Squash	Spinach
Shallots	Potatoes	Pomegranate	Plums
Peas	Pears	Peaches	Oranges
Onions	Nectarines	Mushrooms	Melons
Limes	Lettuce	Lemons	Leafy greens
Kiwi	Green beans	Grapes	Figs
Fennel	Eggplant	Dates	Cucumbers
Cherries	Celery	Carrots	Cabbage
Brussels sprouts	Broccoli	Berries (all types)	Bell peppers
Beets	Bananas	Avocado	Asparagus
Artichokes	Apples		

CHAPTER 5: HOW TO SUCCEED ON THE MEDITERRANEAN DIET

Changing your diet can be quite a challenge, especially if you are adopting one that's very different from yours. Here are tips to make your transition to the Mediterranean Diet easier.

Taste Every Flavor

More than a diet, the Mediterranean diet is a lifestyle that teaches you to enjoy and savor all the flavors of the food you eat. Avoid eating in front of the television since it will take your attention away from the food you are eating. Don't swallow everything in one bite. Instead, eat slowly, take your time, and taste every flavor. Eating slow will also tune your body with the food you eat. Enjoying your meals will even make you eat until you are just satisfied, and a prevent overeating.

Know Your Ideal Weight

Let the ideal weight for your height be your guide. Maintaining your weight gain is essential for good health. If you are overweight, then you need to exercise more and reduce the amount of food you eat and drink. Most people on a diet obsessively count calories, which can distract anyone from enjoying meals. Counting calories also do not work well in the long run.

Be with People You Love

This Mediterranean diet is also based on the principles of enjoyment and pleasure. As much as possible, eat with friends and family. The happy company of others makes the food taste even better, and the laughter you share makes life even better.

Choose a Healthy Lifestyle

Your overall health will not only depend on a healthy eating habit. Together with the Mediterranean diet, exercise and regular physical activities are also important. It doesn't have to be a workout in the gym. It could be as simple as taking the stairs instead of the elevator. Leisurely activities, such as walking, housework, or yard work are also good ways to move your body. You can even do running, aerobics, and other strenuous exercises.

Moderation is the Key

Unlike many diets that involve eliminating certain foods, the Mediterranean diet is a balanced diet that accommodates a wide range of drinks and food. The key is to eat moderately and wisely. On this diet, you can enjoy a small-sized slice of cake, a couple of slices of steak, and 1 to 2 glasses of wine.

Follow the recommended food frequency and portion size

This ensures that you get the right amount of food according to the ones that you can eat in large amounts and more frequently, as well as the those you need to eat in small quantities and less often.

Hydrate

The body is made up of 70 percent water, and proper hydration is essential to maintain energy levels, health, and well-being. Even mild dehydration will affect the processes in your body. The differences in metabolic rates, activity levels, and body type mean that some people need to drink more water than other people.

Eat Eggs

They are excellent sources of high-quality protein and are valuable for people who do not eat meat or vegetarian. Be sure to follow the recommended portions and frequency.

Reduce Salt Intake

Use more herbs and spices and herbs to add flavor and aroma to food instead of salt. They add that distinct Mediterranean cuisine taste and are rich in antioxidants.

Drink Moderately

Follow the recommended daily serving for each type of alcohol. Wine specifically had blood thinning effects, which makes the arteries less prone to clotting. They also contain antioxidants, which help prevent the build-up of low-density lipoprotein, or LDL in the arteries, in turn, avoiding the build-up of plaque in the arteries.

Snack on cheese, low-fat dairy, seeds, and nuts

A handful of sunflower seeds, almonds, and walnuts make great meals. They are portable and on-the-go. Low-fat, calcium-rich cheese and fresh fruits are also great snacks on the go.

Fruits for Dessert

Most fruits are rich in antioxidants, fiber, and vitamin C. They are the healthiest desserts that will satisfy your sweet tooth. Discover and try out new fruits each week and widen your choices.

Increase Whole-Grain Food

It will take some time for your taste buds and stomach to adjust to whole-wheat and whole grain. Slowly replace your refined grain products with whole-grain ones. You can use whole-grain pasta blends or rice. You can also try mixing whole-grains with refined grained, half white and half whole-wheat. When your body has adjusted, then you can switch to whole-wheat and whole-grain completely.

Pack Your Meals with Veggies

Most people do not consume enough veggies. Eat at least 3 to 4 servings a day. The more colorful, the better; more color means more vitamins and minerals. You can add them to your soups and omelets, enjoy them as a vegetable salad, or just roast them.

Switch Proteins

Swapping read meat with turkey, chicken, and fish lowers intake of saturated fat. You can also get your protein from beans, nuts, and other plants. Bream, herring, sardines, tuna, and salmon are good choices. Crustaceans and shellfish, including mussels, shrimps, and clams are also good sources.

Here's a quick way to reduce reduce your meat consumption – make pasta and veggies the star of your meals and use meat as a flavoring or a condiment. Follow the recommended portion size for red meat. On the Mediterranean diet, shellfish and fish are rarely battered or fried.

Use Plant Oils

Use them as your primary fat for cooking and baking. Eliminate all hydrogenated oils and oils containing trans-fat. As much as possible, replace butter and margarine with olive oil and other healthy oils, such as canola, soy, and peanut oil.

For a delicious yet healthy dipping for bread, season high-quality olive oil with balsamic vinegar. When cooking, do not let your oil get to smoking-hot because it will damage their nutritional properties and flavor. There are many interesting variations and many characteristics of olive oil in the market, so experiment to find out which ones you can add to your diet.

Are you ready to start?

CHAPTER 5: 14-DAY MEDITERRANEAN DIET MEAL PLAN

Start your Mediterranean diet journey and taste all the wonderful flavors of the region. Here is a 2-week meal plan to enjoy.

Week 1

Day 1

Breakfast: Fluffy Pancakes

Lunch: Chickpea Salad

Snack: Hummus Crackers with Plum

Dinner: Chicken Kabobs

Day 2

Breakfast: Granola Yogurt Parfait

Lunch: Vegetable Pot Pie – heated 1 Swanson's Chicken Pot or Amy's Vegetable Pot Pie following the package directions.

Serve with 10 pieces of grape tomatoes.

Snack: Creamy Chickpea Spread

Dinner: Tomato and Mozzarella Sandwich

Day 3

Breakfast: Goat Cheese and Chive Frittata

Lunch: Artichoke and Turkey Sandwich

Snack: Creamy Chickpea Spread – reserved spread from Day 2 Snack. Bring 1 cucumber, sliced, for dipping.

Dinner: Grilled Mediterranean Sea Bass PLUS 1 frozen bag of fruit juice (limit the calories of the bar to 80)

Day 4

Breakfast: One serving Fluffy Pancakes (leftover from Day 1 Breakfast) drizzled with 2 tablespoons of light maple syrup. Serve with 1 cup of fat-free milk and 1 One-half cup raspberries.

Lunch: Grilled Mediterranean Sea Bass (reserved Day 3 Dinner) over the reserved leaves of baby arugula.

Snack: Sweet & Sour Cream Dip and Vegetables

Dinner: Baklava and Frittata from Day 3 Breakfast. Eat with 2 cups of baby spinach drizzled with 2 tablespoons 2 tablespoons of balsamic vinegar, 1 slice bread (whole-wheat) spread 2 teaspoons of light margarine (trans-fat-free), and 1 cup milk, fat-free. For dessert, enjoy 1 piece square baklava, about 2-inch (you can eat 2 squares if using Frozen Athens Brand Baklava Pastry).

Day 5

Breakfast: Crunchy and Creamy Yogurt

Lunch: Vegetable Pita Sandwich and Greek Yogurt Cucumber Sauce

Snack: Sweet & Sour Cream Dip (reserved from Day 4 Snack) and Crackers (6 pieces 2 1/2-inch squares of graham crackers, any flavor you desire).

Dinner: Sweet & Sour Mediterranean Chicken

Day 6

Breakfast: Chocolate Milk and Bagel with Peanut Butter

Lunch: Salad and Pizza

Snack: Pineapple Orange Smoothie

Dinner: Greek Cuisine Restaurant – Order lamb or chicken Souvlaki at a Greek restaurant. Eat a bar-soap-sized or 4 ounces lamb or chicken and baseball-sized of couscous rice. Eat all the veggies served with your meal. If served with a salad, drizzle with 1 tablespoon dressing. Pack the leftover lamb or chicken and couscous for Day 7 Lunch, and serve with 2 ounces or half glass of wine.

Day 7

Breakfast: Ricotta Spread Pita and Raisins

Lunch: Souvlaki Lamb (bar-soap-sized or 4 ounces) with couscous or rice (baseball-size or half a cup) from Day 6

Dinner. Serve over 1 cup of cooked spinach or 2 cups of baby spinach.

Snack: Goodie Smoothie - 1 smoothie (Yoplait Nouriche)

Dinner: Shrimp and Basil Summer Salad

Week 2

Day 1

Breakfast: Creamy Ricotta Pancakes

Lunch: Corn, Black Bean, and Tomato Salsa Salad

Snack: Nutty Yogurt

Dinner: Greek Salad and Grilled Chicken

Day 2

Breakfast: Wheat Toast and Western Scrambled Eggs

Lunch: Veggie Burger and New Potatoes

Snack: Yogurt with Pecans and Raisin Bran

Dinner: Crumbled Ground Beef with Tomato Couscous, and Asparagus

Day 3

Breakfast: Energy Bar

Lunch: Heat-and-Serve Italian and Tomatoes

Snack: Veggies and Flavored Hummus

Dinner: Grilled Snapper or Halibut

Day 4

Breakfast: Cherries and Cereal

Lunch: Tuna Pasta

Snack: Crackers, Peanut Butter, and Milk

Dinner: Italian Restaurant - Order chicken Piccata or chicken Marsala. Eat bar-of-soap-sized piece together with a house salad drizzled with 2 teaspoons of olive oil and vinegar or 2 tablespoons full-fat dressing. Enjoy with a side order of pasta (eat One-half cup pasta with sauce) OR with 1 palm-sized slice Italian bread topped with a teaspoon butter. Enjoy 4 ounces wine. Share leftovers with a friend.

Day 5

Breakfast: Smoothie and Cheese

Lunch: Breakfast Dish for Lunch

Snack: Chive and Sour Cream Spread with Veggies

Dinner: Feta Spinach Flatbread

Day 6

Breakfast: One serving Fluffy Pancakes – Reheat the set aside fluffy pancakes from Week 1 Day 1 Breakfast. Top with a mixture of One-third cup sour cream (fat-free) and 1 tablespoon light maple syrup, and 1 cup fresh raspberries. Enjoy with 1 cup milk, fat-free.

Lunch: Feta Cheese Scrambled Eggs

Snack: Peanut Butter and Apple

Dinner: Orzo and Scallops

Day 7

Breakfast: Blueberry and Ricotta Cheese Mixture

Lunch: Lunch Ala Sub Shop

Snack: Sweet & Sour Cream Spread with Vegetables and Fruits

Dinner: Mediterranean-Style Roasted Vegetables

CHAPTER 4: BREAKFAST RECIPES

Fluffy Pancakes

Serves: 5 (4 small-sized pancakes each serving)

Ingredients:

- ½ cup yogurt, low-fat, any flavor

- 1 large-sized egg

- 1 cup buckwheat or whole-wheat pancake mix

Directions:

1. Combine all of the elements until well mixed. Cook the pancakes following the instructions on the pancake mixture package.

2. Enjoy 1 serving or 4 pancakes now and individually pack the remaining 4 servings in the freezer for future meals.

3. Serve pancakes with 2 tablespoons of light maple syrup with a side of 1 of cup fresh strawberries and 1 cup of fat-free milk.

Granola Yogurt Parfait

Serves: 1

Ingredients:

- 6 ounces fruit-flavored light yogurt

- 1 cup raspberries

- 2 tablespoons low-fat granola

Directions:

1. In a wide-mouth, clear glass put 1/3 of the yogurt, 1/3 of the fruit, and then 1/3 of the granola.

2. Repeat the layers until all the ingredients are used. Enjoy!

Goat Cheese and Chive Frittata

Serves: 2

Ingredients:

- 2 whole eggs

- 4 egg whites

- 1/4cup milk

- 1/4 teaspoon salt

- Pinch of ground black pepper

- 1/2 medium-sized tomato

- 1 tablespoon fresh chives, chopped

- 1 teaspoon olive oil

- 1/4 package goat cheese

- 1 cup milk, fat-free, for serving

Directions:

1. Preheat the oven to 375F.

2. In a medium bowl, using a fork or wire whisk, mix the milk, whole eggs, egg whites, pepper, and salt. Stir in the chives and tomato.

3. In an oven-safe 10-inch skillet, heat the olive oil. Pour the egg mixture into the skillet. By spoonfuls, drop goat cheese on top of the egg mixture. Cook for about 3-4 minutes or until the edges of the frittata starts to set.

4. Transfer the skillet to the preheated oven and bake for about 9-10 minutes or until the frittata starts to set ad a knife comes out clean when inserted in the center.

5. Serve half of the frittata. Save and refrigerate the other half for Day4 Dinner.

6. Enjoy your breakfast with 1 cup of fat-free milk.

Crunchy and Creamy Yogurt

Serves 1:

Ingredients:

- 6 ounces of light yogurt, any flavor

- 1 cup high-fiber cereal, such as Kashi Good Friends (or use any cereal – make sure you limit to 100 calories, such as a heaping One-half cup of Raisin Bran or 1 cup cheerios

- 3 tablespoons of chopped walnut

Directions:

1. Put the yogurt in your desired container. Top with your preferred cereal and the walnuts. Enjoy!

Bagel with Peanut Butter and Chocolate Milk

Serves: 1

Ingredients:

- 1 tablespoon peanut butter

- 1-ounce whole-wheat bagel (half of a 170-calorie bagel)

For serving:

- 1 cup milk, fat-free mixed

- 2 teaspoons chocolate syrup

- 1 cup green or red grapes

Directions:

1. Spread the butter on the bagel half.
2. Stir the syrup into the glass of milk until well mixed.
3. Serve the bagel with the chocolate milk and grapes.

Ricotta Spread Pita and Raisins

Serves: 1

Ingredients:

- 1 piece 6 1/2-inch whole-wheat pita

- One third cup ricotta cheese, fat-free

- 1 tablespoon peanut butter

- 1 tablespoon honey

Directions:

1. Mix the cheese with the honey and peanut butter until combined.

2. Fill the pita with the cheese mixture.

3. Add the raisins to the pita mixture.

Creamy Ricotta Pancakes

Serves: 1

Ingredients:

- 1 serving Fluffy Pancakes (leftover from Day 1 Breakfast)

- One-third cup fat-free ricotta cheese

- 1 tablespoon light maple syrup

- 2 tablespoons light maple syrup, for drizzling

For serving:

- 1 cup milk, fat-free

- 1 small-sized orange

Directions:

1. Mix the cheese with a tablespoon of light maple syrup. Layer the pancakes with a spread of the creamy ricotta between each pancake. When the pancakes are layered, drizzle the top with light maple syrup.

2. Serve with 1 cup milk and 1 small-sized orange.

Wheat Toast and Western Scrambled Eggs

Serves: 1

Ingredients:

- 2 egg whites PLUS 1 egg, OR one-fourth cup egg substitute

- 1/2 any color bell pepper, chopped

- One-fourth cup onion, chopped

- Black pepper, to taste

For serving:

- 1 slice bread, whole-wheat, toasted

- 2 teaspoons margarine, trans-fat-free

- 1 cup milk, fat-free

Directions:

1. Scramble the egg and egg white or egg substitute with the rest of the ingredients.

2. Serve the scramble with trans-fat-free margarine topped toasted whole-wheat and milk.

Energy Bar

Serves: 1

Ingredients:

- 1 Luna bar (any kind)

- 8 pieces of pecan halves

- 1 fresh plum

- 1 cup milk, fat-free

Directions:

1. Enjoy!

Cherries and Cereal

Serves: 1

Ingredients:

- 100 calories worth of your favorite cereal (One-half cup raisins and nuts cereal and 1 cup plain flake cereal)

- 1 cup milk, fat-free

- One-half cup fresh cherries, pitted (about 12 pieces)

- 1 stick string cheese

Directions:

1. Put your cereal into a bowl. Pour in the milk and add the cherries.
2. Serve with string cheese.

Smoothie or Jamba Juice

Serves: 1

Ingredients:

- 16-ounce of Enlightened Smoothie or Jamba juice

If you can't find Jamba juice:

- 1/2 teaspoon vanilla

- 1 cup milk, fat-free

- 1 cup strawberries or raspberries

Directions:

1. Enjoy a smoothie or Jamba juice with string cheese.

Blueberry and Ricotta Cheese Mixture

Serves: 1

Ingredients:

- 1 piece (6 1/2-inch) pita, whole-wheat, cut into halves, use 1 half now and save the other half for Day 7 Dinner

For dipping:

- One-half cup ricotta cheese, fat-free

- 1 tablespoon honey

- 3/4 cup fresh blueberries

For serving:

- 1 cup milk, fat-free

Directions:

1. Toast the pita half and then cut into triangles or break into small-sized pieces for dipping.
2. Mix the dipping ingredients until well combined.

3. Scoop the dip with toasted pita pieces.

4. Serve with milk.

Chapter 5: Lunch Recipes

Chickpea Salad

Serves: 1

Ingredients:

- 7 1/2 ounces canned chickpeas (from a 15 ounces can)

- One-fourth cup white onion, chopped, save the piece for dinner

- One-fourth cup green pepper, chopped, save the piece for dinner

- 2 teaspoons of olive oil

- 1 tablespoon black olives, sliced

- 1/4 teaspoon black pepper

- 1 1/2 tablespoons of white vinegar

- 2 cups of romaine lettuce

Directions:

1. Put the canned chickpeas in a colander and rinse under running water for 2 minutes to remove excess sodium. Drain well, set aside and save half of the peas for Day 2: Snack.

2. Except for the romaine lettuce leaves, combine the rest of the ingredients in a bowl until well mixed.

3. Serve over a bed of romaine lettuce leaves.

Artichoke and Turkey Sandwich

Serves: 1

Ingredients:

For the sandwich:

- 2 slices whole-wheat bread

- 1 tablespoon of light mayonnaise

- 4-6 artichoke hearts

- One-third cup 33% reduced-fat mozzarella cheese, shredded

- 3 ounces turkey breast, sliced

For serving:

- 1 cup red or green grapes

- 15 baby carrots

Directions:

1. Spread 1/2 tablespoon light mayonnaise on each whole-wheat bread slice. Stuff the turkey breasts,

mozzarella cheese, and artichoke hearts between the bread.

2. Serve with the grapes and carrots.

Vegetable Pita Sandwich and Greek Yogurt Cucumber Sauce

Serves: 1

Ingredients:

- One-half cup yogurt, plain light

- 1/2 cucumber, finely chopped

- 1/2 garlic clove, minced

- Salt & pepper, to taste

- 1 piece 6 1/2- inch pita, whole-wheat

- 5 grape tomatoes, halved

- 1 cup of string beans

- 1 cup (around 23 pieces) fresh cherries, for serving

Directions:

1. Mix the first 3 ingredients until combined, seasoning with salt and pepper, if desired. Spread 1/2 of the

sauce on the pita pocket. Fill the pocket with the
beans and tomatoes.

2. Serve with the cherries.

Salad and Pizza

Serves: 1

Ingredients:

- 1 slice cheese pizza, large-sized, thin-crust, with vegetable toppings - peppers, onion, and mushrooms

- 2 cups green salad, or more

- 2 tablespoons of regular dressing

For dessert:

- 1 scoop ice cream in a plain cone

Directions:

1. Serve the pizza with the green salad drizzled with the dressing of your choice.
2. Follow with ice cream.

Corn, Black Bean, and Tomato Salsa Salad

Serves: 1

Ingredients:

- 3/4 cup canned black beans

- 1 red tomato, diced

- 1 cooked ear of corn

- 1/2 teaspoon dried basil

- Shake of ground black pepper

- 2 tablespoons of balsamic vinegar

- 1 teaspoon olive oil

For serving:

- 2 cups romaine lettuce

- One third cup 33% reduced-fat mozzarella cheese, shredded

- 1 One-half cups raspberries

Directions:

1. Put the black beans in a colander and rinse under running water to remove excess sodium.
2. Combine the black beans with the rest of the ingredients until well mixed, scraping the corn kernels from them into the mixture.
3. Top the salsa over a bed of romaine lettuce and then top with the shredded cheese.
4. Serve the salad with the raspberries.

Veggie Burger and New Potatoes

Serves: 1

Ingredients:

- 1 vegetable burger of your choice
- 4 small-sized grilled new potatoes (from Day 1 Dinner)
- One-fourth cup shredded cheese
- 2 tablespoons ketchup, optional
- 2 teaspoons spicy mustard, optional

For serving:

- 2 cups leaves baby spinach
- One-fourth cup onion, chopped
- 1/2 bell pepper, cut

Directions:

1. Heat the grilled potatoes and the veggie burger.

2. Top the veggie burger with the cheese and toast in an oven toaster at 250F for about 2 minutes or until the cheese melts.

3. If desired, top the burger with ketchup and spicy mustard.

4. Serve the heated veggie burger and potatoes with the spinach leaves topped with the bell pepper and onion.

Heat-and-Serve Italian and Tomatoes

Serves: 1

Ingredients:

- 1 Healthy Choice Grilled Basil Chicken, OR Spaghetti with Meat Sauce, OR Fettuccine Alfredo

- 15 pieces of grape tomatoes

For dessert:

- 6 ounces of light yogurt, any flavor

- 1 fresh peach

Directions:

1. Heat the Grilled Basil Chicken and serve with the tomatoes.

2. For dessert, enjoy peach dipped in yogurt.

Tuna Pasta

Serves: 1

Ingredients:

- 1 cup cooked whole-wheat pasta, any shape

- 3 ounces white tuna, from can, drained

- 1 1/2 tablespoons light mayonnaise

- Sprinkle of ground black pepper

- One-fourth cup bell pepper, chopped

- One-fourth cup onion, chopped

- 1 fresh plum, for serving

Directions:

1. Except for the plum, combine all of the ingredients.
2. Serve with the plum.

Breakfast Dish for Lunch

Serves: 1

Ingredients:

- 2 slices whole-wheat bread

- 2 tablespoons confectioner's sugar

- 1 cup or baseball-sized fruit salad

Directions:

1. Order from your favorite family-style restaurant or dinner. Ask for whole wheat bread sprinkled with confectioner's sugar and a side of fruit salad in the portions and sizes indicated in the ingredients.

Feta Cheese Scrambled Eggs

Serves: 1

Ingredients:

- 1 egg PLUS 2 egg whites, OR one-fourth cup of egg substitute

- Black pepper, to taste

- 2 tablespoons milk, fat-free

- 2 tablespoons feta cheese, reduced-fat

- Nonstick spray

For serving:

- 2-ounce bagel, whole-wheat

- 1 tablespoon light margarine, trans-fat-free

- 1 cup of spinach greens

- Splash balsamic vinegar

Directions:

1. Whisk the eggs with the black pepper and milk.

2. Grease a skillet with the nonstick spray.

3. Pour the egg mixture. Scatter the cheese over the top of the egg mixture and cook to desired doneness.

4. Serve with bagel spread with margarine and spinach drizzled with balsamic vinegar.

Lunch Ala Sub Shop

Serves: 1

Ingredients:

- 6-inch sub on wheat bread or honey wheat

- Roast beef, ham, turkey, or chicken breast

- 1 tablespoon of light mayonnaise and spicy mustard

- Veggies, such as onion, lettuce, cucumber, tomato, and green pepper

- Baked potato chips (Lay's barbecue or baked Lay's)

- Diet soda

Directions:

1. Get your lunch from the Subway. Choose the ingredients indicated above, leaving the cheese out. Enjoy!

CHAPTER 6: SNACKS

Crackers and Dip

Serves: 1

Ingredients:

- 2 tablespoons hummus

- 1 Wasa Crispbread

- 1 fresh plum

Directions:

1. Spread the hummus over the cracker.
2. Enjoy with fresh plum.

Creamy Chickpea Spread

Serves: 2

Ingredients:

For the spread:

- 7 1/2 ounces chickpeas, saved from Day 1 Lunch

- 2 teaspoons of olive oil

- 1 garlic clove, minced

- 1 tablespoon of lemon juice

- 1/4 teaspoon salt

- 1/4 teaspoon of ground cumin, optional

For dipping:

- 1 cup broccoli florets

- 1 red, yellow, orange bell pepper, sliced

Directions:

1. Prepare the spread in advance. Take half for Day 2 Snack and save the remaining half for Day 3 Snack.

2. Put the chickpeas into a bowl. Using a fork, lightly mash.

3. Add the rest of the ingredients and mix until the spread reaches your desired smoothness. If desired, blend ingredients using your food processor.

4. Put in a container with a tight cover and bring to work along with the broccoli florets and slices of bell pepper.

Sweet & Sour Cream Dip and Vegetables

Serves: 1

Ingredients:

- One-half cup fat-free sour cream (from an 8-ounce pack)

- 1 tablespoon light maple syrup

- 1/4 teaspoon vanilla extract

For dipping:

- 1 cup fresh string beans

- 10 grape tomatoes

Directions:

1. Mix all of the ingredients for the dip. Serve with the beans and tomatoes.

Notes: Reserve the remaining sour cream for Day 5 Snack.

Pineapple Orange Smoothie

Serves: 1

Ingredients:

- One-half cup pineapple chunks, canned and drained or fresh

- 1/2 fresh orange

- 6 ounces light yogurt

Directions:

1. Put all of the ingredients into a blender or food processor, adding ice cubes until the mixture reaches your desired consistency.

2. Serve right away.

Nutty Yogurt:

Serves: 1

Ingredients:

- 6 ounces light yogurt, any flavor

- 3 tablespoons walnuts, chopped

- One-half cup blueberries

Directions:

1. Top the yogurt with the walnuts and blueberries. Enjoy!

Yogurt with Pecans and Raisin Bran

Serves: 1

Ingredients:

- 6-ounces light yogurt

- One-fourth cup raisin bran

- 8 pieces pecan halves

Directions:

1. Serve the yogurt with the pecan halves and raisin bran.

Veggies and Flavored Hummus

Serves: 1

Ingredients:

- 15 pieces baby carrots

- 1 cup string beans

- One-fourth cup hummus, flavored or plain

For serving:

- One-fourth cup soy nuts

Directions:

1. Serve the hummus with the string beans and baby carrots as dipping.
2. Enjoy with soy nuts.

Crackers, Peanut Butter, and Milk

Serves: 1

Ingredients:

- 4 reduced-fat Triscuits, OR 1 Wasa crispbread cracker, OR 2 Ak-Mak crackers

- 1 tablespoon peanut butter

- 1 cup milk, fat-free

Directions:

1. Spread the butter over the crackers.
2. Serve with milk.

Chive and Sour Cream Spread with Veggies

Serves: 1

Ingredients:

- One-half cup fat-free sour cream

- 1 tablespoon dried chives

- 1 garlic clove, minced

For dipping:

- 1 any color bell pepper, sliced

- 1/2 sliced zucchini

Directions:

1. Combine all of the spread ingredients until well combined.

2. Serve with the veggies for dipping.

Peanut Butter and Apple

Serves: 1

Ingredients:

- 1 apple, sliced

- 1 tablespoon of peanut butter

For serving:

- 1 cup milk, fat-free

- 2 teaspoons of chocolate syrup, OR 1 tablespoon strawberry drink mix

Directions:

1. Spread peanut butter on apple slices.
2. Serve with a glass of milk mixed with chocolate syrup or strawberry drink mix.

Sweet & Sour Cream Spread with Vegetables and Fruits

Serves: 1

Ingredients:

- One-half cup sour cream, fat-free

- 1-2 packets Sweet 'N or Low Equal

- 1/4 teaspoon vanilla extract

For dipping:

- 1 One-half cups fresh strawberries, sliced

- 15 grape tomatoes

Directions:

1. Mix the sour cream with the sweetener and vanilla extract. Serve with the strawberries and grape tomatoes.

Chapter 7: Dinner Recipes

Chicken Kebabs

Serves: 1

Ingredients:

- 4 ounces chicken breast, raw, sliced into small-sized chunks

- One-fourth cup Italian dressing, fat-free

- One-fourth cup white onion, saved from Day 1 Lunch

- One-fourth cup green pepper, saved from Day 1 Lunch

- 10 grape tomatoes

- 1 piece -6-inch whole-wheat pita

- 2 tablespoons hummus

Directions:

1. Put the chicken chunks in a bowl. Add the Italian dressing and toss to coat well. Transfer the bowl in

the fridge and let marinate for at least 30 minutes or overnight.

2. Slice the saved green pepper and white onion into chunks.

3. Wash and clean the cherry tomatoes.

4. Alternate the cherry tomatoes, green pepper, white onion, and marinated chicken on skewers and grill until the chicken is cooked.

5. When the kebabs are grilled, grill the pita until toasted. Brush the toasted pita with 2 tablespoons hummus.

6. Serve the kebab with the pita and strawberry milk popsicle (see deserts).

Tomato and Mozzarella Sandwich

Serves: 1

Ingredients:

- 1 piece 6-inch French baguette roll (3-inch diameter)

- One-third cup 33% reduced-fat mozzarella cheese, shredded

- 2 large-sized red tomatoes

- Dried oregano and dried basil, for sprinkling, optional

Directions:

1. In a lengthwise manner, slice the French baguette into halves. Divide the cheese between the two halves, sprinkling it over the cut sides.

2. Put the bread in a toaster oven and bake at 250F for about 4-6 minutes or until the cheese is just starting to melt.

3. Meanwhile, slice the tomatoes into 1/2-inch round slices.

4. Remove the toasted baguette from the oven. If desired, sprinkle with dried oregano and dried basil. Top with the sliced of tomatoes. Serve.

5. Serve with reserved 1 strawberry milk popsicle for dessert.

Grilled Mediterranean Sea Bass

Serves: 2

Ingredients:

- plus 1/2 lemon

- 1 1/2 tablespoons olive oil

- 1/2 tablespoon fresh oregano leaves, chopped

- 1/2 teaspoon ground coriander

- 1/2 plus 1/4 teaspoon salt

- 1 whole sea bass

- 1/8 teaspoon ground black pepper

- 1 large-sized oregano sprig

For serving:

- 1/2 bag of baby arugula, save the remaining half for Day 4 Lunch

- 1 ear corn

- 1 cup sugar snap peas, cooked

- 2 teaspoons trans-fat-free light margarine

Directions:

1. Preheat a gas grill or prepare a charcoal fire for covered direct grilling on medium heat.

2. Meanwhile, from 1 lemon, grate 1 tablespoon of peel and squeeze 2 tablespoons juice. Cut half of the 1/2 lemon into wedges and the other half into slices.

3. In a small-sized bowl, stir the coriander, chopped oregano leaves, olive oil, lemon peel and juice and 1/4 teaspoon of salt.

4. Rinse the sea bass and pat dry using paper towels. Using a sharp knife, cut 3 slashes on both sides of the fish.

5. Sprinkle the outside and inside of the fish with pepper and remaining salt. Put the oregano sprigs and lemon slices inside the fish cavity.

6. Put the fish in a 9x13-inch glass baking dish. Rub the outsides of the fish with 1/2 of the olive oil mixture. Let the fish stand for 15 minutes at room

temperature. Reserve the remaining olive oil mixture for drizzling over the cooked fish.

7. Lightly grease the grill rack and put the fish on the hot tray. Cover and grill the fish for about 12-14 minutes or until the fish is cooked and opaque throughout. The fish is done when the thickest part easily flakes when tested using a fork. Turn the fish once during grilling.

8. To serve, put the fish on a cutting board. Using a knife, moving from head to tail, cut along the backbone of the fish. Slide a full cake server or metal spatula under the front section of the top fillet and lift from the spine. Transfer to a serving plate.

9. Gently pull out the rib bones and backbone from the remaining fillet. Discard the bones. Transfer the bottom fillet to a container with cover and reserve for Day 4 Lunch.

10. Drizzle both of the fillets with the remaining olive oil mixture. Serve the top fillet with lemon wedges. Refrigerate the bottom fillet.

11. Serve the fillet with the baby arugula.

12. Toss the corn and sugar snap peas with the margarine and serve on the side.

13. Enjoy 1 frozen fruit juice bar for dessert.

Sweet & Sour Mediterranean Chicken

Serves: 1

Ingredients:

- 1/4 teaspoon olive oil

- 2 small-sized chicken thighs, skinless

- 1/16 teaspoon salt

- 1/2 clove garlic

- 1/8 cup chicken broth

- 1/8 cup red wine vinegar

- 1/4 teaspoon cornstarch

- 1/4 teaspoon brown sugar

- 3/16 cups Mission figs

- 1/16 cups salad olives

- ¼ bag baby arugula

Directions:

1. Put the olive oil in a nonstick skillet and heat. When the oil is hot, add the chicken and sprinkle with salt; cook for about 17-20 minutes or until is browned meat juices of the thickest part run clear when pierced with the tip of a knife. Turn the chicken once during cooking.

2. Meanwhile, in a cup, mix the sugar, cornstarch, vinegar, and broth using a wire whisk.

3. When the chicken is cooked, transfer the chicken to a plate.

4. Add the garlic to the skillet; sauté for 30 seconds.

5. Stir the broth mixture and then add into the skillet; heat until boiling and boil for 1 minute, stirring to loosen the browned bits from the bottom of the skillet, until the sauce is slightly thick. Stir in the olives and the figs.

6. Return the chicken to the skillet and heat through.

7. To serve, arrange the arugula on a dinner plate and spoon the chicken mixture over the arugula.

8. Serve with One-half cup of cooked brown rice topped with 2 teaspoons of light margarine (trans-fat-free)

9. Enjoy 4 ounces of wine!

Shrimp and Basil Summer Salad

Serves: 1

Ingredients:

- 9 large-sized or 12 medium-sized shrimp (about 3 ounces)

- 2 cups romaine lettuce

For the basil marinade:

- One-fourth cup white wine vinegar

- 1 teaspoon olive oil

- 1 tablespoon of lemon juice

- 1 teaspoon dried basil or 1/8 cup fresh basil, chopped

Directions:

1. Whisk together the marinade ingredients until combined. Toss the shrimp with the marinade and let marinate for at least 30 minutes or overnight.

2. Grill the shrimp until cooked through.

3. Arrange 2 cups romaine lettuce. Put the grilled shrimp on the bed of lettuce and mix into the greens to spread the flavor.

4. Serve with 1 cup blueberries.

5. For dessert, serve remaining strawberry milk popsicle.

Greek Salad and Grilled Chicken

Serves: 1

Ingredients:

- 3-ounce of chicken breast

- 3 tablespoons Italian dressing, fat-free

- 9 small-sized new potatoes

- Olive oil cooking spray

- Dash black pepper

For serving:

- One and one-half cups of romaine lettuce

- 1 tablespoon black olives, sliced

- One-half ounce feta cheese, reduced-fat, crumbled

For the dressing:

- 1/2 teaspoon of dried basil

- 2 teaspoons of olive oil

- 1/2 teaspoon dried basil

- 1 garlic clove, minced

- Couple shakes black pepper

Directions:

1. Marinate the chicken with the Italian dressing for at least 30 minutes or overnight. Spray the potatoes with the olive oil and sprinkle with the black pepper.

2. Grill the chicken and the potatoes until cooked.

3. Serve 5 of the grilled potatoes now and reserve 4 for Day 2 Lunch.

4. Whisk all of the dressing ingredients until combined.

5. Arrange the romaine lettuce on a plate, top with the olives, feta cheese and drizzle with the dressing.

6. Serve the chicken and potatoes with the salad.

Crumbled Ground Beef with Tomato Couscous, and Asparagus

Serves: 1

Ingredients:

- 2 ounces of dry couscous

- 4 ounces ground beef patty, 90%-92% lean

- 10 spears of asparagus

- Nonstick olive oil cooking spray

- Three-fourth cup jarred spaghetti sauce

For serving:

- 4 ounces of wine

Directions:

1. Cook the couscous according to the directions on the package.

2. Grease the beef patty and asparagus with the olive oil and grill until cooked to desired doneness.

3. When cooked, crumble the beef patty into the cooked couscous. Chop the asparagus spears and add to the mixture.

4. Top with the spaghetti sauce and serve with wine.

GRILLED SNAPPER OR HALIBUT

Serves: 2

Ingredients:

- 1/2 of an onion, sliced into round slices

- 1 can (8-ounce) diced tomatoes (with no added salt)

- 12 ounces red snapper or halibut

For serving:

- 1 cup of brown rice, cooked (One-half cup per serving)

For dessert:

- Frozen bar fruit juice (limit amount of calories to 90)

Directions:

1. Fashion a sturdy 10-inch diameter bowl from several pieces of aluminum foil, folding the edges up a bit.

2. Put the diced tomatoes in the aluminum foil bowl. Put the red snapper or halibut on top of the tomatoes.

Grill until the fish is cooked or easily flakes when tested using a fork. Grill the sliced onions alongside the fish and tomatoes until cooked.

3. Divide the grilled fish, tomatoes, and onion over brown rice. Serve.

4. Enjoy a frozen fruit juice bar for dessert.

Feta Spinach Flatbread

Serves: 1

Ingredients:

- 1 piece 6 1/2-inch pita bread, whole-wheat

- 3/4 cup leaves baby spinach

- 2 tablespoons feta cheese, reduced-fat

- 1 scallion, chopped

- 1/2 teaspoon lemon juice

- Black pepper, to taste

- Nonstick cooking spray, for cooking the pita

For serving:

- 2 cups of spinach leaves

- One-eighth cup red onion, chopped

- One-fourth cup zucchini, diced

- 2 tablespoons dressing, full-fat

- 2 tablespoons pine nuts, toasted

For dessert:

- Chocolate popsicle, see recipe

Directions:

1. Open the pita bread, layer the rest of the ingredients inside the pita pocket.
2. Grease a nonstick skillet with the cooking spray.
3. Put the pit I the skillet and grill each side for 2 minutes.
4. Serve with the spinach leaves topped with the rest of the ingredients for serving.
5. Enjoy a chocolate popsicle for dessert.

Orzo and Scallops

Serves: 1

Ingredients:

- 2/3 cup of cooked orzo

- 1/2 of a red onion, sliced, save the remainder for Day 7 Dinner

- 1/2 of an eggplant, sliced, keep the rest for Day 7 Dinner

- 16 scallops

For the marinade:

- One-fourth cup Italian or Tuscan-style salad dressing

- One-half cup of apple juice

For serving: 4 ounces wine

Directions:

1. Cook the orzo according to package directions.

2. Mix the marinade ingredients. Divide into two portions. Save 1 portion for basting the scallops.

3. Put the scallops in the remaining marinade and let marinate for 30 minutes.

4. After marinating, discard the scallop marinade.

5. Grill the veggies until cooked, basting with the reserved marinade.

6. Grill the scallops for about 2 minutes each side and brush with the reserved marinade.

7. Top the orzo with the grilled veggies and scallops.

8. Enjoy with wine!

Mediterranean-Style Roasted Veggies

Serves: 2

Ingredients:

- 1 zucchini, sliced

- 2 any color bell peppers, sliced

- Remaining veggies from Week 2 Day 6 Dinner (one-half red onion and one-half eggplant), sliced

- 1 tablespoon of olive oil

- 2 tablespoons hummus

- 1-2 teaspoons of dried oregano

- 1/2 teaspoon salt

- Shake of black pepper

Directions:

1. Put the veggies in foil. Drizzle with the olive oil and season with the salt, dried oregano, and black pepper.

2. Completely wrap the foil around the veggies. Grill for about 10 minutes each side.

3. Serve with the remaining pita half from Day 7 Breakfast. Grill the pita for about 1-2 minutes and spread with the hummus.

Chapter 8: Desserts

Strawberry Milk Popsicle

Serves: 3

Ingredients:

- 1 cup milk, fat-free

- 1 tablespoon strawberry drink mix

Directions:

1. Put the milk in a large-size glass and stir in the strawberry drink mix.

2. Pour the mixture into 3 pieces popsicle molds and freeze overnight. You can serve the popsicles as a healthy dessert. Serve 1 and save the remaining 2 popsicles for Day 2 and Day 7 desserts.

Chocolate Popsicle

Serves: 3

Ingredients:

- 8 ounces fat-free milk

- 2 teaspoons chocolate syrup

Directions:

1. Mix the milk and chocolate syrup until well combined.

2. Pour into 3 popsicle molds and freeze until frozen.

Final Words

Thank you again for purchasing this book! I really hope this book is able to help you.

The next step is for you to **join our email newsletter** to receive updates on any upcoming new book releases or promotions. You can sign-up for free and as a bonus, you will also receive our "*7 Fitness Mistakes You Don't Know You're Making*" book! This bonus book breaks down many of the most common fitness mistakes and will demystify many of the complexities and science of getting into shape. Having all this fitness knowledge and science organized into an actionable step-by-step book will help you get started in the right direction in your fitness journey! To join our free email newsletter and grab your free book, please visit the link and signup: **www.hmwpublishing.com/gift**

Finally, if you enjoyed this book, then I would like to ask you for a favor, would you be kind enough to leave a review for this book? It would be greatly appreciated!

Thank you and good luck in your journey!

About the Co-Author

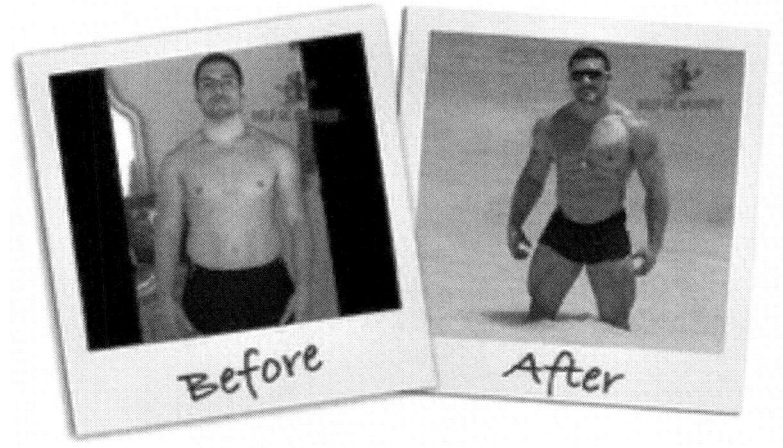

Before After

My name is George Kaplo; I'm a certified personal trainer from Montreal, Canada. I'll start off by saying I'm not the biggest guy you will ever meet and this has never really been my goal. In fact, I started working out to overcome my biggest insecurity when I was younger, which was my self-confidence. This was due to my height measuring only 5 foot 5 inches (168cm), it pushed me down to attempt anything I ever wanted to achieve in life. You may be going through some challenges right now, or you may simply want to get fit, and I can certainly relate.

For me personally, I was always kind of interested in the

health & fitness world and wanted to gain some muscle due to the numerous bullying in my teenage years about my height and my overweight body. I figured I couldn't do anything about my height, but I sure can do something about how my body looked like. This was the beginning of my transformation journey. I had no idea where to start, but I just got started. I felt worried and afraid at times that other people would make fun of me for doing the exercises the wrong way. I always wished I had a friend that was next to me who was knowledgeable enough to help me get started and "show me the ropes."

After a lot of work, studying and countless trial and errors. Some people began to notice how I was getting more fit and how I was starting to form a keen interest in the topic. This led many friends and new faces to come to me and ask me for fitness advice. At first, it seemed odd when people asked me to help them get in shape. But what kept me going is when they started to see changes in their own body and told me it's the first time that they saw real results! From there, more people kept coming to me, and it made me realize after so much reading and studying in this field that it did help me but it also allowed me to help others. I'm now a fully certified personal trainer and have trained numerous clients to date who have achieved amazing results.

Today, my brother Alex Kaplo (also a Certified Personal Trainer) and I own & operate this publishing venture, where we bring passionate and expert authors to write about health and fitness topics. We also run an online fitness website "HelpMeWorkout.com" and I would love to connect with by inviting you to visit the website on the following page and signing up to our e-mail newsletter (you will even get a free book).

Last but not least, if you are in the position I was once in and you want some guidance, don't hesitate and ask... I'll be there to help you out!

Your friend and coach,

George Kaplo
Certified Personal Trainer

Get another book for Free

I want to thank you for purchasing this book and offer you another book (just as long and valuable as this book), "Health & Fitness Mistakes You Don't Know You're Making", completely free.

Visit the link below to signup and receive it:

www.hmwpublishing.com/gift

In this book, I will break down the most common health & fitness mistakes, you are probably committing right now, and I will reveal how you can easily get in the best shape of your life!

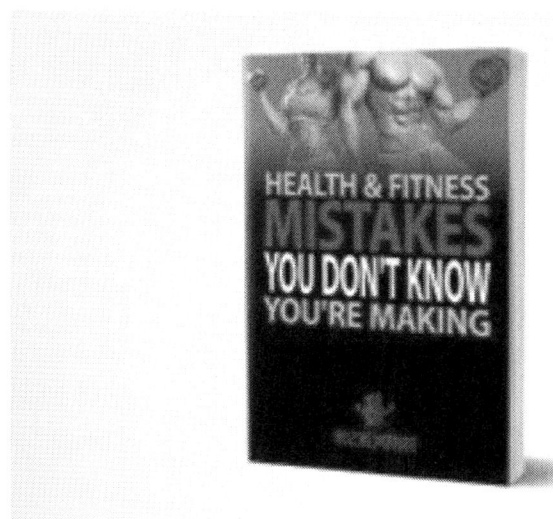

In addition to this valuable gift, you will also have an opportunity to get our new books for free, enter giveaways, and receive other valuable emails from me. Again, visit the link to sign up:

www.hmwpublishing.com/gift

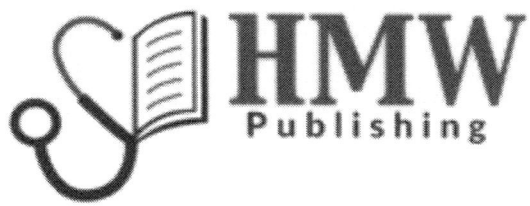

For more great books visit:

HMWPublishing.com

33254044R00088

Printed in Great Britain
by Amazon